COMPLETE GUIDE TO HEMORRHOIDS

The Ultimate Comprehensive Handbook For Immediate Relief, Effective Treatment Methods, And Proven Prevention Strategies

DEHART HAIRSTON

DISCLAIMER

This book's content is only intended for general informative purposes. At the time of writing, the author has taken every precaution to guarantee that the material is correct and current. Nevertheless, the author disclaims all explicit and implicit representations and guarantees about the availability, appropriateness, correctness, completeness, and usefulness of the material on these pages.

Since the author is not a licensed medical practitioner, the material in this book shouldn't be interpreted as medical advice. Before making any modifications to their diet, exercise regimen, or medical treatment, readers are urged to speak with a licensed healthcare provider.

Moreover, the author has no connection to any of the businesses, organizations, or people that are discussed in this book. Any mentions of goods, services, businesses, or people are purely informative and do not indicate endorsement or suggestion.

This book's content is entirely dependent on the author's expertise, study, and comprehension of the topic. Despite having taken reasonable care to offer correct information, the author disclaims all liability for any mistakes or omissions in the material as well as for any losses, harm, or damages resulting from using the information.

It is recommended that readers use their own judgment and discretion when applying the knowledge in this book to their own situations. The use or implementation of any material in this book may result in unfavorable repercussions, directly or indirectly, for which the author assumes no liability.

By reading this book, you agree to release and hold the author harmless from any claims, losses, liabilities, costs, or expenditures resulting from or related to the use of the information you get from it.

Table of Contents

ABOUT THE BOOK

"Hemorrhoids" is an invaluable resource that provides in-depth knowledge about comprehending, treating, and avoiding hemorrhoids. This book, with its well-ordered chapters, is an information source for anybody struggling with this widespread yet sometimes misdiagnosed illness.

Readers will obtain a comprehensive grasp of hemorrhoids, including their numerous forms, underlying causes, and telltale indications and symptoms to look out for, by delving into the foundations in Chapter 1. This basic understanding enables people to identify the problem and take immediate action.

An in-depth discussion of the rectum and anus' anatomy and physiology is provided in Chapter 2, which also highlights the risk factors and the process by which hemorrhoids arise.

With this information at hand, readers may make more educated decisions about their lifestyle and health.

In Chapter 3, which walks readers through recognizing hemorrhoids, knowing when to seek medical assistance, and comprehending diagnostic processes, the need for early diagnosis and assessment is emphasized. Proactive healthcare management and prompt action are encouraged in this area.

Since prevention is usually preferable to treatment, Chapter 4 describes practical methods for preventing hemorrhoids via food changes, lifestyle changes, and good cleanliness. Through the use of these preventive steps, readers may protect themselves from the pain associated with hemorrhoids.

A wide range of therapeutic alternatives, including over-the-counter drugs, home cures, and natural therapies, are provided in Chapters 5 and 6. Whether researching topical treatments or using herbal therapies, readers learn important tips for properly treating hemorrhoids from the comfort of their own homes.

Chapters 7 and 8 explain several therapeutic techniques, such as sclerotherapy, hemorrhoidectomy, and rubber band ligation, for people who need medical intervention. With this information, people may work with their healthcare professionals to make well-informed choices.

Chapter 9 discusses post-treatment care and recovery, highlighting the significance of coping with pain, following through on lifestyle modifications, and guaranteeing a seamless recovery process. Ultimately, Chapter 10 gives readers the tools they need to take control of their health journey by providing advice on maintaining a long-term lifestyle and recurrence prevention techniques.

Essentially, "Hemorrhoids" offers a whole toolset for anybody afflicted with this problem rather than simply a book. By providing readers with information, tactics, and tools, this book turns into a vital tool for managing hemorrhoids and improving general health.

CHAPTER 1

Understanding Hemorrhoids

What Are Hemorrhoids?

Hemorrhoids, sometimes called piles, are enlarged veins in the anus or lower rectum. Many things may cause these veins to swell or become inflamed, which can cause pain, discomfort, and even bleeding when you move your bowels. They may appear outwardly around the anus or inwardly inside the rectum.

Internal hemorrhoids may not be felt or seen; instead, they form within the rectum. Usually, they result in painless hemorrhaging while passing gas. In contrast, external hemorrhoids appear as lumps or bumps under the skin around the anus. They might be painful, and irritating, and cause itching, particularly while you're sitting or having a bowel movement.

Types Of Hemorrhoids

Hemorrhoids come in two primary varieties: internal and external.

Internal hemorrhoids are painless hemorrhoids that form within the rectum. They are usually not felt or seen, although they might cause bleeding during bowel movements. In extreme circumstances, they could poke out of the anus, hurting or irritating others.

External hemorrhoids: These feel like lumps or bumps and develop under the skin surrounding the anus. They may itch, hurt, or make you uncomfortable, particularly if you're sitting or having bowel motions. External hemorrhoids may sometimes develop blood clots that cause thrombosis and excruciating discomfort.

Causes Of Hemorrhoids

Veins in the rectum or anus become enlarged or irritated, leading to hemorrhoids. Hemorrhoids may occur as a result of many factors:

• **Straining during bowel movements:** Pressure from excessive straining during stool passage might cause edema and inflammation in the rectum's veins.

• **Prolonged diarrhea or constipation:** irregular bowel movements might raise the risk of hemorrhoids. Specifically, constipation may make it more difficult to pass feces, which can cause straining and elevated vein pressure.

• **Pregnancy:** Hormonal changes and increased pelvic pressure during pregnancy may aggravate or start hemorrhoids.

• **Obesity:** Being fat or overweight increases the pressure on the veins in the anus and rectum, which increases the risk of hemorrhoids.

• **Extended durations of sitting or standing:** Prolonged sitting or standing may reduce blood flow to the lower abdomen, which can exacerbate hemorrhoids.

• **Genetics:** Certain people may be genetically predisposed to hemorrhoids.

Symptoms And Signs

Hemorrhoids may present with a variety of symptoms, depending on the kind and severity of the ailment. Typical indications and manifestations include:

• **Bleeding during bowel movements:** When hemorrhoids are internal, this is often the first indication of the condition. The blood in the toilet bowl or on the toilet paper may be a vivid crimson color.

• **Itching or irritation:** The area surrounding the anus may become itchy or irritated due to external hemorrhoids.

• **Pain or discomfort:** External hemorrhoids may be painful or uncomfortable, particularly while sitting or having bowel movements.

• **Swelling or lumps:** Around the anus, external hemorrhoids may be felt as soft lumps or bumps. In extreme circumstances, blood clots may develop within external hemorrhoids, resulting in thrombosis—a painful swelling.

• **Prolapse:** Internal hemorrhoids may come out of the anus and then return, particularly when bowel motions are involved.

It's essential to comprehend these indications and symptoms to spot hemorrhoids early and get the right care. A healthcare provider must be consulted to get an accurate diagnosis and a customized treatment plan.

CHAPTER 2

Anatomy And Physiology

The Anatomy Of The Rectum And Anus

Comprehending the development of hemorrhoids and the variables that contribute to their occurrence requires an understanding of the anatomy of the rectum and anus. The rectum, which connects the colon to the anus, is the last segment of the large intestine, measuring about 15 cm in length. It acts as a holding area for feces before their expulsion from the body. The orifice where feces leaves the body after the digestive system is called the anus.

Hemorrhoids develop and function because of several important structures located in the rectum and anus. These consist of muscular tissue, blood vessels, and connective tissues that sustain them. The real hemorrhoids are composed of groups of blood vessels and surrounding tissue in the anal canal, and they are a typical anatomical feature. By assisting in the closure of the anus, they help regulate the amount of stool produced.

Changes in blood vessel pressure may happen in the rectum and anus, especially while straining during bowel motions, sitting or standing for extended periods, or moving heavy objects. Hemorrhoids may result from an enlargement or inflammation of these veins.

How Hemorrhoids Develop

When the blood vessels in the rectum or anus enlarge or become irritated, hemorrhoids occur. This swelling may be seen externally, around the anus entrance, or internally, inside the rectum. Hemorrhoids come in two primary varieties: internal and external.

Because there are fewer pain-sensing nerves in the rectum, internal hemorrhoids usually cause no discomfort. On the other hand, they could result in pain, itching, or bleeding during bowel movements. External hemorrhoids, which occur around the anus opening, maybe more painful, particularly if blood clots (thrombosis) grow inside of them. They may cause itching, inflammation, and pain and can manifest as lumps or bulges around the anus.

Elevated blood vessel pressure in the rectum and anus is often linked to the development of hemorrhoids. There are other potential causes of this pressure, such as:

1. Stifling while passing gas, which may happen when suffering from diarrhea or constipation.

2. Prolonged standing or sitting, which may prevent the flow of blood to the lower abdomen.

3. Being overweight or obese might put more strain on the pelvic floor and lower abdomen.

4. Pregnancy might increase the risk of hemorrhoids by putting extra strain on the pelvic veins.

5. Aging, since the anus and rectum's blood vessel-supporting tissues may deteriorate with time.

People who are aware of these risk factors may be able to lower their chance of hemorrhoids by taking preventative action.

Risk Factors

The risk of hemorrhoids may be raised by several risk factors. These include underlying medical issues as well as lifestyle choices that raise the pressure on the blood vessels in the rectum and anus.

1. Bad Diet: Constipation may result from a low-fiber diet, which can also put strain on the rectum and anus blood vessels and produce discomfort during bowel movements. Consuming a diet high in fruits, vegetables, and whole grains helps lower the incidence of hemorrhoids and encourages regular bowel movements.

2. Sedentary Lifestyle: Being inactive may lead to obesity and constipation, two conditions that increase the risk of hemorrhoids. Frequent exercise may help lessen pelvic floor discomfort and enhance bowel movement.

3. Obesity: Carrying a large weight or being obese puts extra strain on the pelvic veins, which may lead to hemorrhoids. This risk may be decreased by maintaining a healthy weight via food and exercise.

4. Pregnancy: Women who are pregnant are more likely to get hemorrhoids due to hormonal changes and increased strain on the pelvic veins. Furthermore, the stress of giving delivery may increase this risk even more.

By drinking plenty of water, eating a high-fiber diet, and avoiding extended periods of sitting or standing, pregnant women may lower their risk of hemorrhoids.

5. Chronic Constipation or Diarrhea: Irritable bowel syndrome (IBS) and inflammatory bowel disease (IBD) are two conditions that may cause chronic constipation or diarrhea. These conditions put pressure on the rectal region during bowel movements, which can raise the risk of hemorrhoids. To manage these problems and lessen the risk of hemorrhoids, dietary and lifestyle modifications should be made in addition to seeking medical attention when needed.

6. Family History: People who have a family history of hemorrhoids may be more prone to have the problem themselves, suggesting that there may be a genetic predisposition to hemorrhoids. Although genetics cannot be altered, people may lower their risk of hemorrhoids by taking preventative actions after learning about this risk factor.

People may lower their risk of hemorrhoids and improve overall colorectal health by being aware of these risk factors and adopting proactive measures to minimize them. To avoid hemorrhoids and promote normal digestive function, one should adopt several lifestyle practices such as regular exercise, keeping a healthy weight, eating a balanced diet high in fiber, staying hydrated, and practicing excellent personal hygiene.

CHAPTER 3

Diagnosis And Evaluation

Identifying Hemorrhoids

The first step to treating hemorrhoids properly is diagnosing the disease. Swollen veins in the lower rectum and anus that may cause pain, discomfort, itching, and bleeding are called hemorrhoids, or piles. It's essential to identify hemorrhoid symptoms to treat and intervene as soon as possible.

Rectal bleeding is one of the main signs of hemorrhoids, particularly while one is boweling. Depending on how severe the hemorrhoids are, the color of the bleeding might be bright red or darker. Rectal bleeding should never be disregarded since it may be a sign of more severe illnesses including colorectal cancer.

Anal inflammation, pain, and itching are frequent symptoms of hemorrhoids. A sense of fullness or soreness in the rectum may accompany this itching and discomfort. Furthermore, lumps or edema around the anus may sometimes be felt as a result of external hemorrhoids.

Hemorrhoids may prolapse in some situations, meaning that they come out of the anus during bowel movements or other activities. Hemorrhoids that prolapse may hurt and may need to be treated by a doctor.

When To See A Doctor

Although self-care techniques are often effective in managing hemorrhoids, medical assessment and treatment may be required in some cases. To avoid complications and guarantee appropriate treatment of the problem, it is important to understand when to seek medical assistance for hemorrhoids.

It is imperative that you see a doctor right away if you have severe or ongoing rectal bleeding. Hemorrhoids are one of the many reasons for rectal bleeding, but they may also indicate more severe disorders that need to be treated by a doctor.

In the same vein, you should see a physician for assessment if you have prolonged anal itching, discomfort, or pain. These symptoms may be an indication of hemorrhoids or other rectal diseases that need to be treated, and they may have a major negative influence on your quality of life.

It is imperative that you get medical assistance if you discover any lumps or swelling around the anus, particularly if they are uncomfortable or sensitive. These might be indicators of external hemorrhoids or other illnesses that need to be assessed and treated by a medical expert.

Diagnostic Procedures

Hemorrhoids are usually diagnosed by a combination of physical examination, medical history, and sometimes further diagnostic tests. Although physical examination results and symptoms are often used to identify hemorrhoids, there are times when further testing is necessary to confirm the diagnosis or rule out other possible causes.

Your doctor will visually examine the rectum and anus during a physical examination to look for hemorrhoidal symptoms including prolapse, edema, or irritation. A greased, gloved finger is inserted into the rectum to feel for anomalies during a digital rectal examination.

In some instances, your physician could suggest further diagnostic tests, such as anoscopy, sigmoidoscopy, or colonoscopy, to assess the degree and character of the hemorrhoids and exclude any plausible reasons for your complaints. Anoscopy is the process of seeing the lower rectum and anal canal by passing a tiny, tube-shaped device called an anoscope through the anus. The more involved procedures known as sigmoidoscopy and colonoscopy enable visibility of the whole colon and rectum with the use of a flexible, illuminated tube known as a sigmoidoscope or colonoscope.

Based on the degree and scope of your hemorrhoids, these diagnostic techniques may assist your doctor in determining the best course of therapy. They may also assist in ruling out more severe illnesses that would call for other treatments.

CHAPTER 4

Prevention Strategies

Lifestyle Modifications

Modifications to your way of living may both relieve the symptoms of hemorrhoids and drastically lower your chance of getting them. Staying physically active regularly is important. Exercise stimulates bowel movements and prevents constipation, which is a major cause of hemorrhoids, thereby promoting good digestion. Simple exercises that increase circulation and lessen strain on the rectal veins include yoga, swimming, and walking.

Avoiding extended periods of standing or sitting is another way to change one's lifestyle. Extended sitting puts pressure on the rectal region, which may result in hemorrhoids. Should your occupation need extended periods of sitting, schedule frequent intervals to stand, stretch, and move about. In a similar vein, consider sometimes raising your legs to increase blood flow if your work requires you to stand.

Preventing hemorrhoids also requires maintaining a healthy weight. Being overweight increases the strain on the abdomen and pelvis, which raises the possibility of hemorrhoids. You may lessen the pressure on your rectal veins by achieving and maintaining a healthy weight with the aid of a balanced diet and frequent exercise.

Furthermore, maintaining good posture might help avoid hemorrhoids. Hemorrhoids may develop as a result of increased pressure on the rectal region caused by slouching or bad posture while sitting. To properly align your spine and lessen the pressure on your lower back and pelvis, sit up straight with your shoulders back.

Finally, do not postpone having bowel movements. Disregarding the desire to urinate might result in constipation, which raises the possibility of hemorrhoids. Pay attention to your body's cues and act quickly if you sense that you should have a bowel movement.

Dietary Recommendations

One of the most important things in controlling and avoiding hemorrhoids is eating a balanced diet. Maintaining regular bowel movements and avoiding constipation—a major risk factor for hemorrhoids—requires consuming an adequate amount of fiber. Consume a diet high in fruits, vegetables, whole grains, and legumes, among other fiber-rich foods.

In addition, staying hydrated is crucial to avoiding hemorrhoids. Water consumption softens feces, facilitating passage and lowering the risk of constipation.

Try to consume eight glasses of water or more each day, and avoid or limit alcohol and caffeine since they may also lead to dehydration.

Certain meals may aid in promoting good digestion and preventing hemorrhoids in addition to fiber and water. Foods high in probiotics, such as kefir, sauerkraut, and yogurt, have good bacteria that promote gut health and regular bowel motions. Citrus fruits, strawberries, and bell peppers are among the foods strong in vitamin C that help strengthen blood vessels and lower the incidence of hemorrhoids.

However, certain foods and drinks should be restricted or avoided since they may worsen the symptoms of hemorrhoids. Caffeine, alcohol, processed meals, and spicy foods may irritate the digestive system and cause diarrhea or constipation, which both raise the risk of hemorrhoids.

It is recommended to concentrate on a diet high in whole, unprocessed foods and to eat these products in moderation.

Hygiene Practices

Maintaining good cleanliness is crucial to avoiding anal irritation and inflammation, which may worsen the symptoms of hemorrhoids. To prevent inflammation, clean the anal region with simple water or mild, unscented wipes. As strong soaps and wipes with alcohol or scents might aggravate sensitive skin even more, stay away from using them.

Instead of rubbing the anal region dry after bowel movements, since this might irritate it, gently pat it dry with a soft cloth. Steer clear of scratchy toilet paper since this may exacerbate pre-existing hemorrhoids or lead to the development of new ones.

When cleaning, think about utilizing a bidet or moistened wipes for a more thorough and delicate cleaning.

Keeping a clean bathroom and following excellent hygiene practices may also help avoid hemorrhoids. When having a bowel movement, try not to strain since this might put more pressure on the rectal veins and lead to the development of hemorrhoids. Rather, just unwind and let the thoughts come out on their own. If you're worried about constipation, try adding dietary fiber and drinking plenty of water to help encourage softer stools and more easily passed bowel motions.

Lastly, if you already have hemorrhoids, think about using over-the-counter ointments or lotions to reduce discomfort and inflammation. These products usually include hydrocortisone or witch hazel, which are anti-inflammatory and anti-itching agents.

CHAPTER 5

Over-The-Counter Treatments

Topical Medications

One of the most popular over-the-counter remedies for hemorrhoids is topical medicine. These drugs, which are available in cream, ointment, and gel forms, are intended to relieve the burning, itching, and swelling sensations connected to hemorrhoids.

Witch hazel is a natural astringent that may help decrease swelling and relieve pain. It is one of the main constituents in many topical hemorrhoid treatments. Other frequent chemicals include pramoxine, which temporarily relieves itching and pain, and hydrocortisone, which helps decrease inflammation.

It's crucial to carefully follow the directions on the label while using topical drugs. Generally, depending on how severe your symptoms are, you'll apply a tiny quantity of the drug to the afflicted region up to multiple times a day. To stop the transmission of germs, wash your hands both before and after using the drug.

Furthermore, it's crucial to remember that whilst topical treatments may provide momentary relief from hemorrhoid symptoms, they cannot deal with the underlying source of the ailment. You may need to look into other treatment options, such as dietary adjustments or surgical treatments, for hemorrhoids that are more severe or chronic.

Suppositories

Another over-the-counter remedy for hemorrhoids is suppositories. To provide treatment directly to the diseased region, these tiny, bullet-shaped capsules are placed into the rectum. When topical treatments alone are not enough to cure internal hemorrhoids, suppositories are often used to relieve the condition.

Since the drug enters the circulation via the thin lining of the rectum, suppositories have the benefit of offering focused treatment to the root of the issue. This may lead to symptom alleviation from pain, swelling, and itching occurring more quickly.

Hemorrhoid suppositories often include lidocaine, which temporarily relieves discomfort and itching, and hydrocortisone, which helps decrease inflammation. Additionally, some suppositories may include natural substances like aloe vera or witch hazel, which may help relieve sensitive skin.

It's crucial to carefully follow the directions on the label while using suppositories. Depending on the severity of your symptoms, you will usually inject one suppository into the rectum up to multiple times each day. To stop the transmission of germs, make sure you wash your hands both before and after using them.

Suppositories may not be appropriate for everyone, even though they may effectively relieve hemorrhoid symptoms. Before using suppositories to treat your hemorrhoids, you should speak with your doctor if you have any underlying medical issues or are on any drugs.

Sitz Baths

Hemorrhoid pain may be effectively and simply relieved with Sitz baths. This entails spending many minutes each day, for fifteen to twenty minutes at a time, sitting in a warm, shallow bath. Warm water relieves pain and irritation by reducing swelling and soothing inflamed skin.

You may either fill a bathtub with a few inches of warm water or use a specifically made sitz bath basin that fits over the toilet to take a sitz bath. To further relieve the afflicted region, you may also add items to the water, including baking soda or Epsom salts.

Making sure the water is not too hot is crucial while having a sitz bath since this might aggravate the skin even more. Additionally, because strong cleansers and soaps may dry out the skin and make symptoms worse, you should avoid using them.

Use a fresh towel to gently pat the region dry after a sitz bath. For further relief, you may also apply a calming lotion or ointment to the afflicted region. Sitz baths may be used as often as necessary to help relieve the symptoms of hemorrhoids.

By increasing blood flow to the damaged region, sitz baths may aid in healing in addition to relieving symptoms. This may help you feel more like yourself again sooner by lowering inflammation and accelerating the healing process.

CHAPTER 6

Home Remedies

Natural Remedies

Even though they are unpleasant, hemorrhoids are often successfully treated using natural therapies that capitalize on the properties of natural components. Witch hazel, a natural astringent with anti-inflammatory qualities, is one such treatment. Using a cotton ball to apply witch hazel to the afflicted region will help relieve itching and pain and decrease swelling.

Aloe vera, which has healing and calming qualities, is another natural cure. Direct application of aloe vera gel to the hemorrhoids might aid in reducing swelling and accelerating recovery. Using pure aloe vera gel without any other components is crucial since it might hurt the delicate skin around the anus.

Hemorrhoid symptoms may also be relieved by taking an Epsom salt bath. Soaking for 15 to 20 minutes in warm bath water with Epsom salts will help minimize soreness and swelling. Additionally, the warm water promotes circulation and muscular relaxation, both of which may speed up recovery.

Herbal Treatments

For millennia, people have utilized herbal remedies to reduce hemorrhoid symptoms and encourage recovery. Horse chestnut, which has ingredients that strengthen blood vessels and lower inflammation, is one well-liked herbal medicine. Horse chestnut may be administered topically as an ointment or lotion, or it can be taken orally as a supplement.

Another plant that's often used to cure hemorrhoids is the butcher's broom. It has ingredients that support blood vessel strength and minimizes edema. You may use a butcher's broom directly to the afflicted region or consume it orally.

Lastly, studies have shown that bilberry extract strengthens blood vessels and improves circulation, suggesting that it may be a useful therapy for hemorrhoids. Supplements containing bilberry extract may be used orally to assist lessen pain and edema.

Home Care Tips

Several home care techniques may help reduce hemorrhoid symptoms and encourage recovery in addition to natural therapies and herbal treatments. One crucial piece of advice is to keep the anal region clean by gently washing it with warm water after bowel movements. Steer clear of strong soaps or wipes since they might irritate delicate skin.

Constipation is a significant cause of hemorrhoids, so eating a high-fiber diet and drinking enough water may also help avoid it. Fiber eases the passage of stool and softens it, which lessens the pressure on the rectum and anus.

Regular exercise and avoiding extended periods of sitting or standing may also assist to enhance circulation and lessen the strain on the veins in the anal region. Use a cushion or pillow in the form of a doughnut to reduce pressure on the hemorrhoids while seated.

Lastly, developing healthy toilet habits may aid in preventing additional discomfort and promoting healing. Examples of these behaviors include not straining during bowel movements and not holding it in when you feel the need to go.

You may efficiently treat hemorrhoids and encourage recovery in the comfort of your own home by implementing these herbal medicines, home care recommendations, and natural cures into your routine. If your symptoms are severe or prolonged, remember to see a healthcare provider since they could need medication.

CHAPTER 7

Medical Treatments

Rubber Band Ligation

Hemorrhoids may be treated medically using rubber band ligation, especially internal hemorrhoids that do not improve with conventional methods. A reasonably easy operation is usually carried out in a physician's office.

This is how it works: the physician will wrap a little rubber band around the root of the hemorrhoid using a specialized instrument. As a result, the hemorrhoid essentially stops receiving blood, shrinking and finally falling off in a matter of days.

The actual process is normally painless, although both during and after the surgery, you can feel some pressure or discomfort. After rubber band ligation, most patients can return to their regular activities right away, however, it's advised to refrain from heavy lifting and vigorous activity for a few days.

The efficiency of rubber band ligation is one of its primary benefits. Research indicates that it is generally effective in treating internal hemorrhoids, with comparatively few side effects. Additionally, the process is really quick—it usually only takes a few minutes to complete.

Sclerotherapy

Another medical treatment for hemorrhoids is sclerosing therapy, which is especially useful for tiny internal hemorrhoids. The hemorrhoid will shrink and finally vanish as a result of the doctor injecting a chemical solution straight into it during this operation.

The operation doesn't need anesthesia and is usually carried out in a doctor's office.

A little burning or stinging sensation may be experienced during the injection, however this normally goes away fast.

Although it may not be appropriate for everyone, sclerosing hemorrhoids is generally seen to be a safe and successful treatment option. Those with lesser hemorrhoids or those who are not suitable candidates for other treatments are often advised to have it.

Sclerotherapy has the benefit of being a reasonably short procedure—it typically takes a few minutes to complete. The majority of individuals may go back to their regular activities right after, however it's advised to refrain from heavy lifting and vigorous activity for a few days.

Infrared Coagulation

Hemorrhoids may be treated non-surgically using infrared coagulation (IRC), which employs heat to reduce the hemorrhoidal tissue. A tiny probe is placed into the rectum during the treatment, and the hemorrhoid is exposed to brief bursts of infrared light, which causes it to contract and finally vanish.

Anesthesia is not needed for IRC procedures, which are usually carried out in a physician's office. Although the actual surgery is normally painless, you can feel warm or uncomfortable in the rectal region.

One benefit of IRC is that it's a really easy and fast process, often just a few minutes to complete. The majority of individuals may go back to their regular activities right after, however it's advised to refrain from heavy lifting and vigorous activity for a few days.

All things considered, IRC is regarded as a secure and successful hemorrhoid treatment approach, especially for minor internal hemorrhoids. It may not be appropriate for everyone, however, so it's crucial to speak with a physician to find the best course of action for your particular circumstances.

CHAPTER 8

Surgical Interventions

When conservative therapy for hemorrhoids is ineffective or the situation is severe, surgical options are usually taken into consideration. We'll look at the many surgical choices in this chapter, such as stapled hemorrhoidopexy, hemorrhoidectomy, and other surgical treatments.

Hemorrhoidectomy

A surgical technique called a hemorrhoidectomy is used to eliminate hemorrhoids. When alternative treatments have failed or for severe instances of hemorrhoids, it is often advised. Hemorrhoidal tissue is incised around by the surgeon, who then excises the enlarged veins during a hemorrhoidectomy. The patient's health and the surgeon's choice will determine whether this treatment is performed under local anesthetic, spinal anesthesia, or general anesthesia.

Patients may feel some pain and discomfort after the surgery; this may be controlled with painkillers that the doctor has given. Patients are recommended to adhere to a particular diet, refrain from straining during bowel movements, and use stool softeners to prevent constipation during the few weeks that follow a hemorrhoidectomy.

Hemorrhoids may be effectively treated with a hemorrhoidectomy, but there are risks and consequences involved, such as infection, bleeding, and trouble urinating. As a result, before making a choice, people should talk with their doctor about the procedure's possible dangers and advantages.

Stapled Hemorrhoidopexy

Hemorrhoids may be treated using a minimally invasive surgical surgery called stapled hemorrhoidopexy, often referred to as stapled hemorrhoidectomy or procedure for prolapse and hemorrhoids (PPH). Using a specialized tool known as a stapler, the surgeon performs this operation to remove extra tissue and realign the hemorrhoids.

Because stapled hemorrhoidectomy causes less discomfort and requires a quicker recovery than standard hemorrhoidectomy, it is often favored. Most patients can return home the same day or the day following surgery, even though the treatment is done under general anesthesia.

Although stapled hemorrhoidopexy is typically safe, not all patients will benefit from treatment, particularly if they have extensive external hemorrhoids or certain medical disorders.

Although they are uncommon, problems including bleeding, infection, and fecal incontinence are still a possibility.

Other Surgical Options

Depending on the severity of the problem and the demands of the patient, surgical options for treating hemorrhoids may include alternatives to hemorrhoidectomy and stapled hemorrhoidopexy. Among them are:

• **Rubber band ligation:** A technique whereby the physician encircles the hemorrhoid's base with a tiny rubber band to cut off its blood supply, causing it to contract and fall out.

• **Sclerotherapy:** An injection of a chemical solution into the hemorrhoid to cause it to shrink.

• **Coagulation procedures:** Heat is used to shrink the hemorrhoid in techniques like infrared coagulation and laser coagulation.

• **Hemorrhoidal artery ligation:** To decrease blood flow and shrink the hemorrhoid, the surgeon shuts off the blood arteries feeding the tumor.

Patients who choose less invasive therapies or who are not candidates for stapled hemorrhoidectomy or hemorrhoidopexy may be advised to consider these surgical alternatives. To choose the best plan of action for their unique requirements, individuals should, however, go over their alternatives with their doctor.

CHAPTER 9

Recovery And Aftercare

Post-Treatment Care

Following any kind of hemorrhoid treatment—drugs, surgeries, or procedures—it's critical to follow a thorough post-treatment care regimen. This stage is crucial to guaranteeing a speedy recovery and averting recurrences.

Keeping up with cleanliness is a crucial part of post-treatment care. This entails using mild, odorless soap and water or wet wipes to gently clean the anal region after bowel motions. It's critical to stay away from strong or perfumed products to avoid irritation, which may make pain worse.

To facilitate recovery, it's also critical to keep the anal region dry. Wearing breathable cotton underwear and gently patting the region with a soft cloth after cleaning will help avoid moisture accumulation and lower the risk of infection.

For the best possible outcome, it's important to follow any prescription ointments or treatments in addition to good cleanliness. These might be oral drugs to lower inflammation and encourage healing, or local lotions to relieve pain and itching. Effective treatment depends on you adhering to your healthcare provider's dose and application recommendations.

Finally, scheduling regular follow-up visits with your physician is essential in the post-treatment stage. These consultations enable timely resolution of any issues or difficulties, monitoring of your progress, and any required modifications to your treatment plan.

Managing Discomfort

One of the most frequent side effects of hemorrhoid therapy is discomfort. Thankfully, several techniques may ease pain and encourage recovery.

Acetaminophen and ibuprofen are two examples of over-the-counter pain medications that are quite helpful in managing discomfort. These drugs may lessen the discomfort and swelling brought on by hemorrhoids.

Applying ice or cold packs to the anal region in addition to taking medicine will help reduce discomfort and swelling right away. Apply the ice pack to the afflicted region for 10 to 15 minutes at a time, covering it with a cloth or towel to keep it from coming into contact with the skin.

Sitz baths, which include bathing the anal region in warm water for ten to fifteen minutes on many occasions a day, may also aid in easing pain and accelerating the healing process. By calming sensitive skin, adding Epsom salts to the water may provide extra comfort.

Moreover, maintaining healthy bowel habits might aid in preventing pain from becoming worse. To encourage regularity and soften stools, this involves avoiding straining during bowel movements, drinking enough of water, and eating a high-fiber diet.

Lifestyle Adjustments

Modifying one's lifestyle is crucial to keeping anal health generally and avoiding hemorrhoids from recurring.

A healthy, high-fiber diet is one of the most important lifestyle changes. Constipation is a major risk factor for hemorrhoids and may be avoided by consuming fiber, which also helps to encourage regular bowel movements.

Consume a diet rich in fruits, vegetables, whole grains, and legumes to guarantee that your consumption of fiber is sufficient.

Moreover, softening stools and avoiding constipation depends on remaining hydrated throughout the day by consuming plenty of water. Try to consume eight glasses of water or more each day, and avoid or limit alcohol and caffeine since they may also lead to dehydration.

Exercise regularly is also essential for preserving anal health. Engaging in physical exercise may enhance colon health and circulation, which lowers the chance of hemorrhoids. Most days of the week, try to get in at least 30 minutes of moderate activity, such as cycling, swimming, or walking.

Finally, minimizing extended periods of sitting or standing may help minimize pressure accumulation in the anal region, which lowers the chance of hemorrhoids. If your work needs you to sit for extended periods, take regular breaks to stand and stretch. You may also want to use a donut pillow or cushion to ease pressure on your anal area. In the same vein, attempt to shift your weight often and take brief sitting breaks whenever you can if you must stand for lengthy periods.

By implementing these lifestyle changes into your everyday routine, you may help keep your anals at their best and stop hemorrhoids from recurring. Before making any big dietary or activity changes, remember to speak with your doctor, particularly if you have any underlying medical concerns.

CHAPTER 10

Lifestyle Maintenance

Long-Term Strategies

Long-term successful hemorrhoid management requires maintaining a healthy lifestyle. A balanced diet, consistent exercise, and healthy bowel practices are all part of this.

Diet: To avoid constipation, which may worsen hemorrhoid symptoms, a high-fiber diet is crucial. Fruits, vegetables, whole grains, legumes, and other high-fiber foods encourage regular bowel movements and soften feces, making them easier to pass without straining. It's crucial to maintain proper hydration, so make sure you sip plenty of water all day long.

Exercise: Getting regular exercise increases circulation and helps to boost bowel movement, both of which may lower the incidence of hemorrhoids. Aim for at least 30 minutes of moderate exercise most days of the week. Walking, swimming, and cycling are all fantastic options.

Steer clear of straining: straining during bowel movements may place too much pressure on the veins in the lower abdomen, which can exacerbate or cause hemorrhoids. Refrain from sitting on the toilet for extended periods, and do not push stools through if they are not ready to pass.

Keep Your Weight in Check: Being overweight or obese may aggravate symptoms and raise the risk of hemorrhoids. To lessen the tension in the rectal region, maintain a healthy weight via food and exercise.

Good Bowel Habits: Constipation and straining may be avoided by developing regular bowel habits. Aim for a daily bowel movement around the same time, ideally just after eating when the gastric reflex is at its highest. Don't postpone having bowel movements and use the restroom as soon as you sense the need.

Avoid Extended Sitting or Standing: Prolonged sitting or standing might put more strain on the veins in the lower abdomen. Take regular pauses to stretch and move about if your profession demands you to sit or stand for extended amounts of time.

Preventing Recurrence

Effective hemorrhoid management may alleviate symptoms, but it's crucial to take precautions against recurrence.

Maintain Healthy Habits: To avoid further flare-ups, keep up the healthy lifestyle practices mentioned above even after hemorrhoid symptoms have decreased. Long-term management requires consistency.

Handle Stress: Stress may aggravate digestive problems, such as constipation and diarrhea, which can lead to the emergence or recurrence of hemorrhoids. Engage in hobbies and enjoyable activities, deep breathing exercises, mindfulness, meditation, and other stress-reduction strategies.

Prevent Straining During Bowel Movements: One of the main causes of hemorrhoids is straining during bowel movements. Make sure you eat a lot of fiber, drink enough water, and have regular bowel movements to avoid constipation and lessen the need to strain.

Be Aware of cleanliness: Having good cleanliness will help avoid anal irritation and infection, both of which can exacerbate hemorrhoid symptoms. Use mild, unscented toilet paper or moist wipes to gently clean the anal region after bowel movements.

Steer clear of abrasive soaps or wipes that include alcohol or smell since they may irritate the skin.

Don't Ignore Symptoms: Be mindful of any modifications in your bowel patterns or any symptoms, including discomfort, bleeding, or itching in the rectal region. See your doctor for further assessment and treatment if you have severe or recurring symptoms.

Regular Check-ups: Make an appointment for routine check-ups with your physician, particularly if you've previously had hemorrhoids or other gastrointestinal problems. They can keep an eye on your health and provide advice on ways to lower the chance of a relapse.

When To Seek Further Medical Advice

Even though lifestyle changes and over-the-counter medications may often successfully control hemorrhoids, there are certain situations in which further medical counsel or intervention may be required.

Persistent Symptoms: It's crucial to see your doctor for further assessment if you continue to have symptoms like bleeding, itching, or discomfort even after changing your lifestyle and using over-the-counter medications.

Severe Symptoms: You may need to see a doctor if you have severe symptoms including heavy bleeding, excruciating pain, or prolapsed hemorrhoids, which occur when internal hemorrhoids push outside the anus. Your doctor can determine how severe your symptoms are and suggest the best course of action.

Changes in Bowel Habits: Any chronic constipation, diarrhea, or changes in the consistency of your stool may be signs of an underlying gastrointestinal problem that needs to be evaluated by a doctor.

Family History: It's crucial to be on the lookout for any changes in bowel habits or symptoms and to get medical attention right once you have a family history of colorectal cancer or other gastrointestinal disorders.

Medical History: You may be more susceptible to problems from hemorrhoids if you have a history of inflammatory bowel disease, liver illness, or a compromised immune system. For individualized advice on how to manage your illness, speak with your healthcare practitioner.

Pregnancy: Because the pelvic veins are under more strain, hemorrhoids are often seen during pregnancy. For safe and efficient treatment options, speak with your healthcare professional if you are pregnant and suffering from hemorrhoids.

Side effects of medication: Some drugs, such as iron supplements or painkillers, might exacerbate hemorrhoid symptoms and cause constipation. Talk to your healthcare practitioner about any possible adverse effects if you take any drugs that might impair your ability to urinate.

Previous Treatment Failures: It could be time to see a healthcare professional for other treatment choices if you've tried over-the-counter medications or home cures without success. Based on your particular demands, they may evaluate your illness and suggest suitable solutions.

Hemorrhoids may be properly managed and their negative effects on your quality of life reduced by being proactive about maintaining your lifestyle, avoiding recurrence, and recognizing when to seek further medical counsel.

CONCLUSION

In summary, hemorrhoids are a common and often unpleasant medical ailment that millions of people experience globally. Even though they may result in uncomfortable symptoms including discomfort, itching, and rectal bleeding, they are usually treatable with a variety of approaches. By being aware of the risk factors—such as pregnancy, obesity, and persistent constipation—people may lessen their chance of hemorrhoids by taking preventive action.

Hemorrhoids may be treated with anything from simple lifestyle changes like eating more fiber and drinking plenty of water to more intrusive techniques like rubber band ligation or, in extreme situations, surgical removal. However, to get an accurate diagnosis and customized treatment programs, people must speak with healthcare specialists.

In addition, it is possible to mitigate symptoms and prevent recurrence by implementing good behaviors such as eating a balanced diet, exercising often, and avoiding extended sitting or straining during bowel movements. Furthermore, over-the-counter treatments like sitz baths and topical lotions may provide momentary pain alleviation.

Hemorrhoids may sometimes go away on their own without the need for medical attention. On the other hand, to rule out any other possible underlying diseases and to guarantee proper therapy, persistent or severe symptoms call for medical attention.

Additionally, lowering the stigma attached to talking about bowel-related problems and increasing public knowledge about hemorrhoids might motivate people to seek prompt medical attention, improving their quality of life and results.

Hemorrhoids are often curable and managed, even though they may cause pain and inconvenience. People may manage hemorrhoids and lessen their impact on everyday life with the right knowledge, preventative actions, and access to healthcare.

THE END